Kids Yoga Stories'

Good Night, Animal World

A Kids Yoga Bedtime Story

Written by Giselle Shardlow
Illustrated by Emily Gedzyk

Good Night, Animal World

ISBN-13: 978-1492210443
ISBN-10: 1492210447

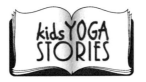

Kids Yoga Stories
Boston, MA
www.kidsyogastories.com
www.amazon.com/author/giselleshardlow
Email us at info@kidsyogastories.com

What do you think?
Let us know what you think of **Good Night, Animal World**
at feedback@kidsyogastories.com.

Printed in the U.S.A.

For my gorgeous parents, who taught my brother and me healthy sleep habits
for life. I am forever grateful for your love and support.
~ G.S. ~

For my mother, who taught me from the start to love all creatures,
big and small.
~ E.G. ~

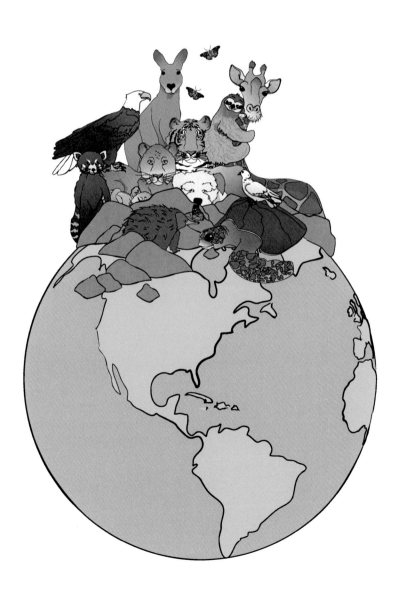

Welcome to a Kids Yoga Stories Bedtime Book

Dear Readers,

Calm your mind and body before bedtime by taking a journey around the world with this kids yoga storybook. Say good night to special animals from six continents: Central America, Asia, Australia, North America, Europe, and Africa.

On every page, one of the six yoga kids will show you the calming yoga pose that corresponds to the animal on each page. The poses are suitable for everyone, even yoginis as small as toddlers and preschoolers. Please also encourage your children to use their imaginations to act out the keywords. Embrace their creativity and let them experiment with the poses. Whatever helps them release extra energy before bedtime is the perfect pose.

The reference guide at the end of this book includes a list of the traditional names of the yoga poses, a map showing each animal on its home continent, and a parent guide with tips on creating a successful bedtime experience.

Enjoy your trip around the world and, as always, be safe. Sleep well.

Love,

Giselle

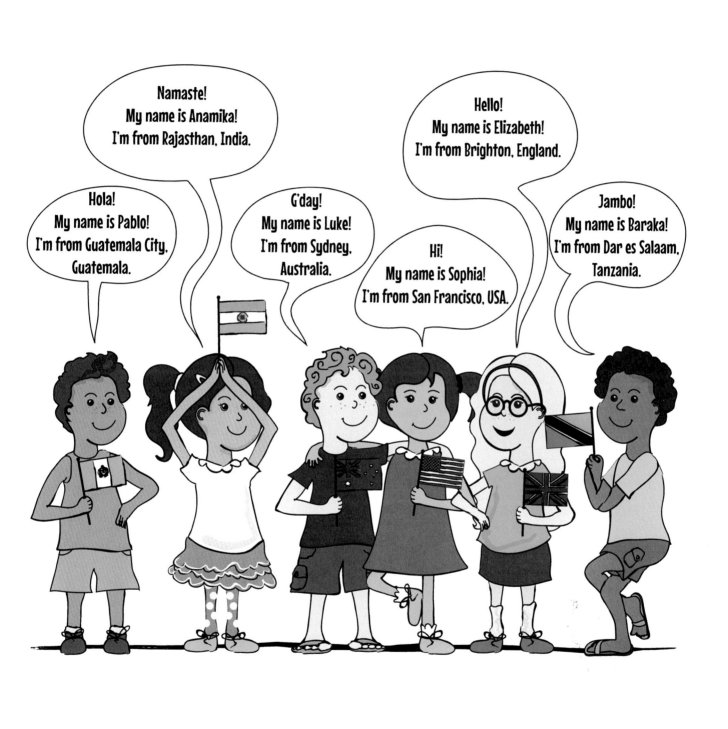

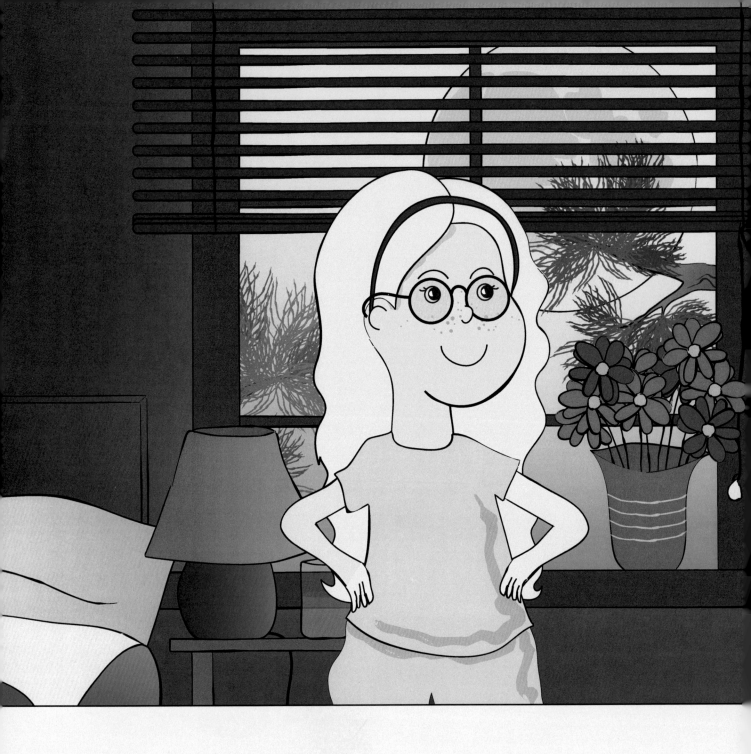

Hello, animals around the world.
It is time to say good night.

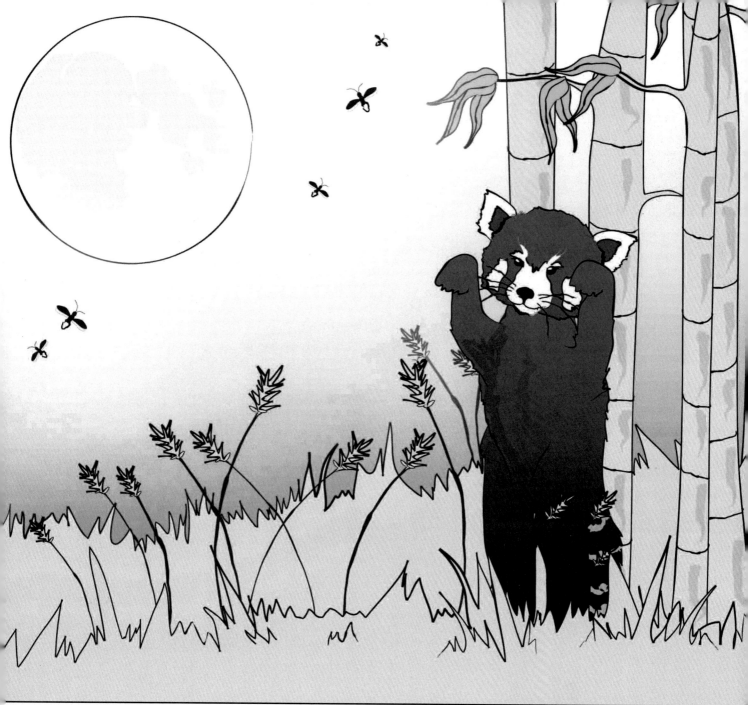

The **panda** is reaching up to the full moon. Good night, panda.

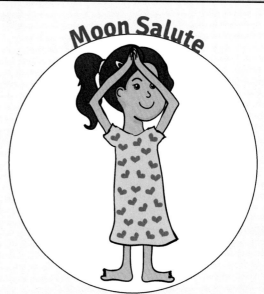

Moon Salute

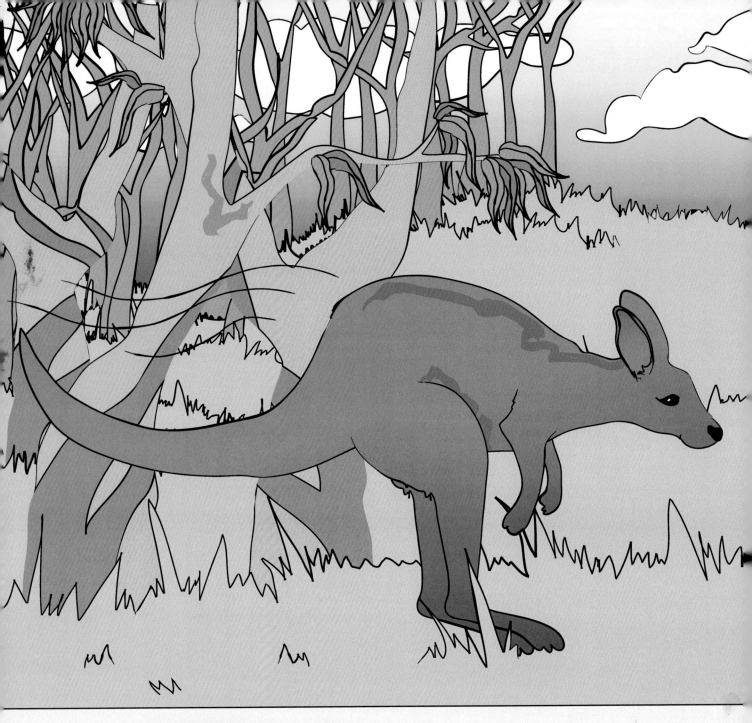

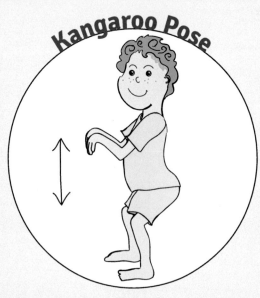

Kangaroo Pose

The **kangaroo** is bounding through the blue gums. Good night, kangaroo.

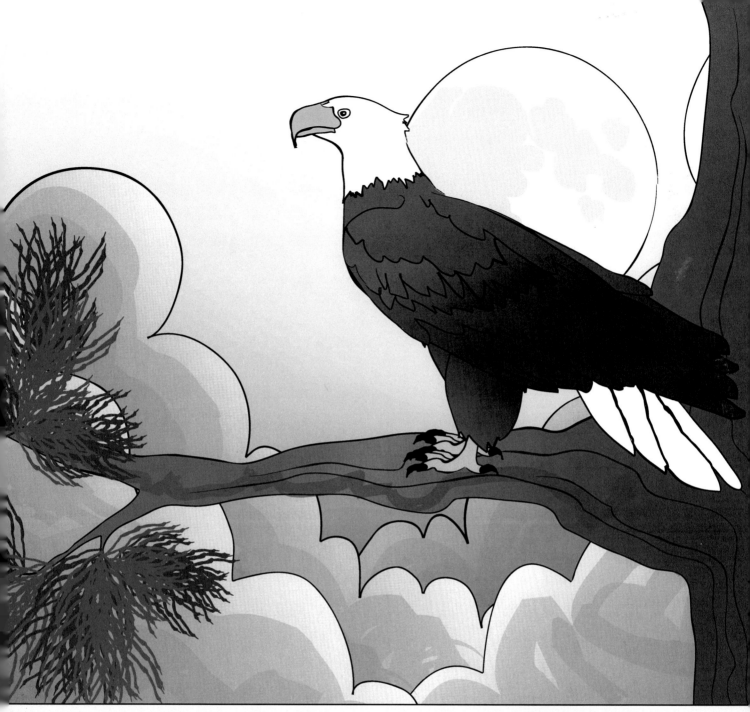

The **eagle** is perched on
a pine tree.
Good night, eagle.

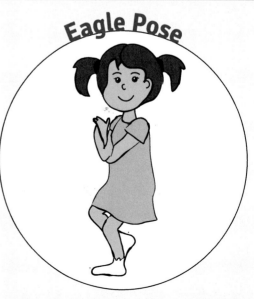

Eagle Pose

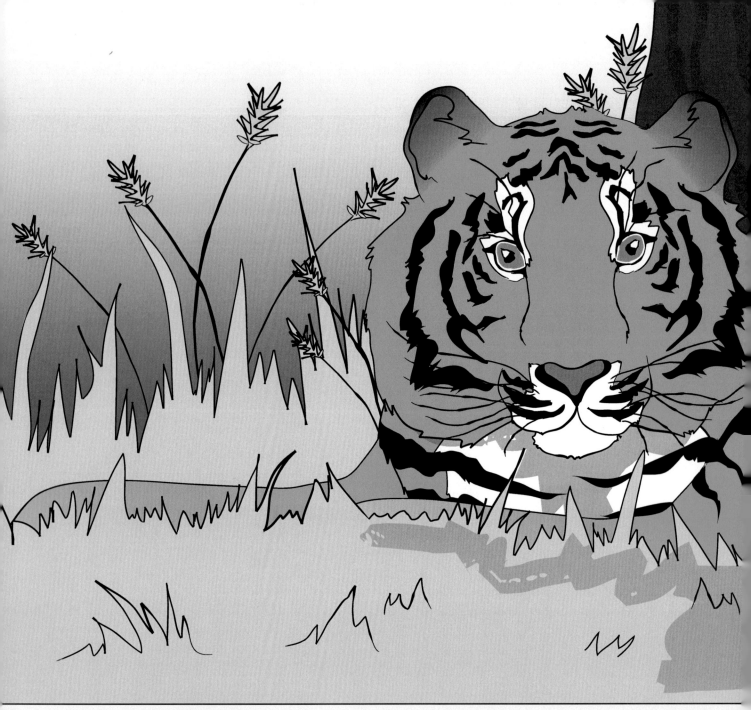

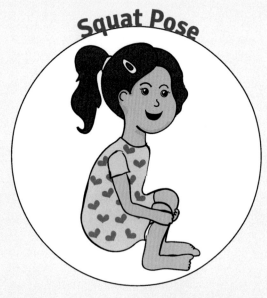

Squat Pose

The **tiger** is crouched in a temperate forest. Good night, tiger.

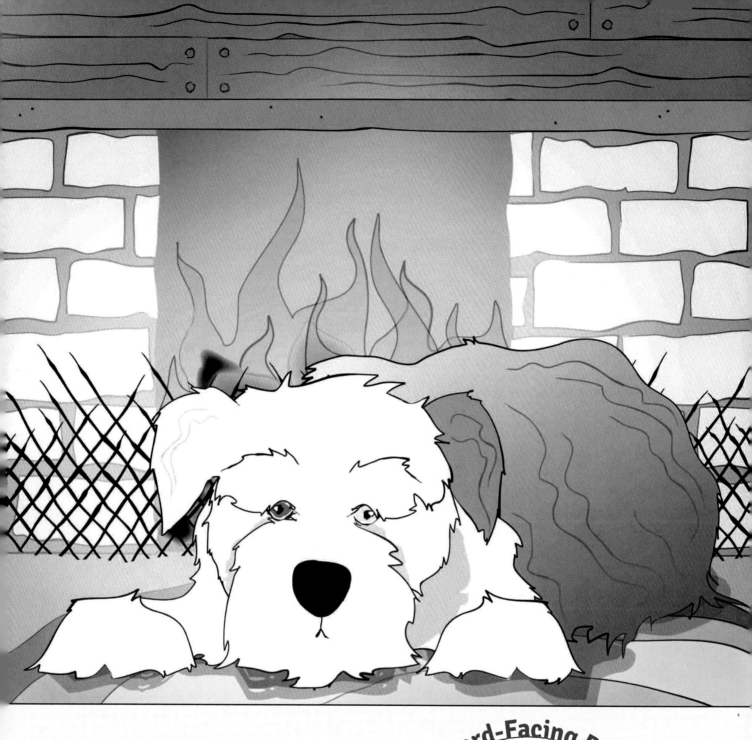

The **sheepdog** is
stretching beside
the warm fire.
Good night, sheepdog.

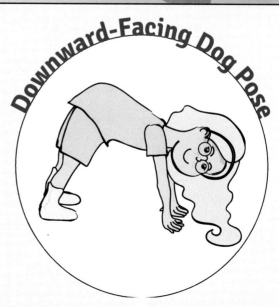

Downward-Facing Dog Pose

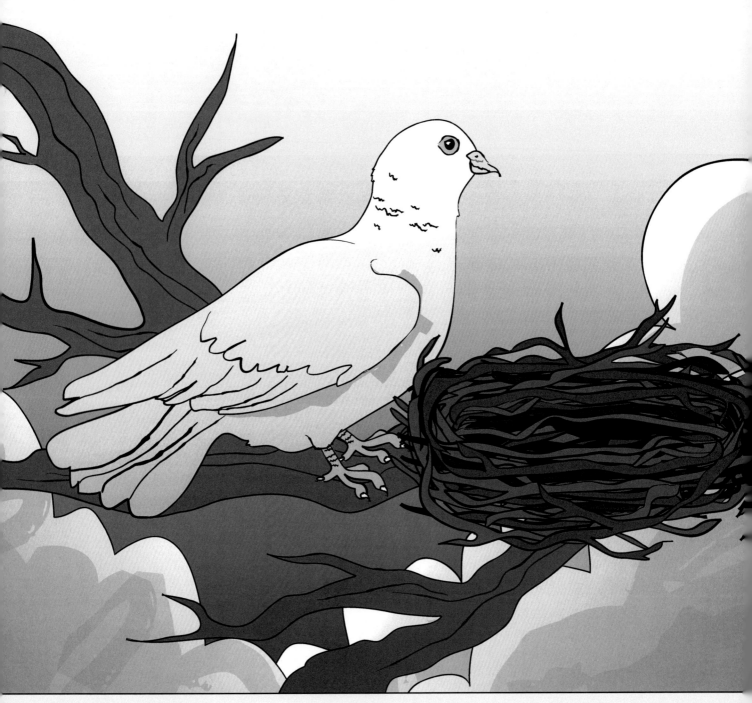

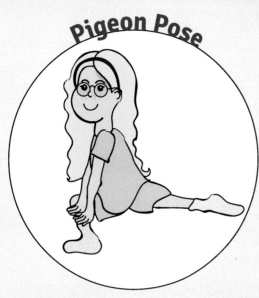

Pigeon Pose

The **dove** is building a nest of twigs.
Good night, dove.

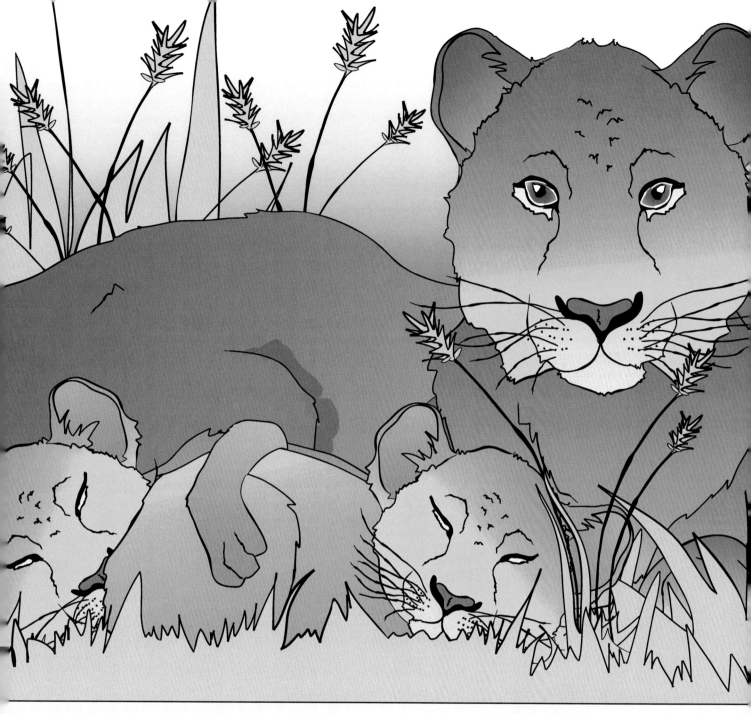

The **lioness** is watching her sleepy cubs.
Good night, lions.

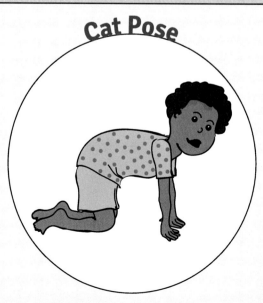

Cat Pose

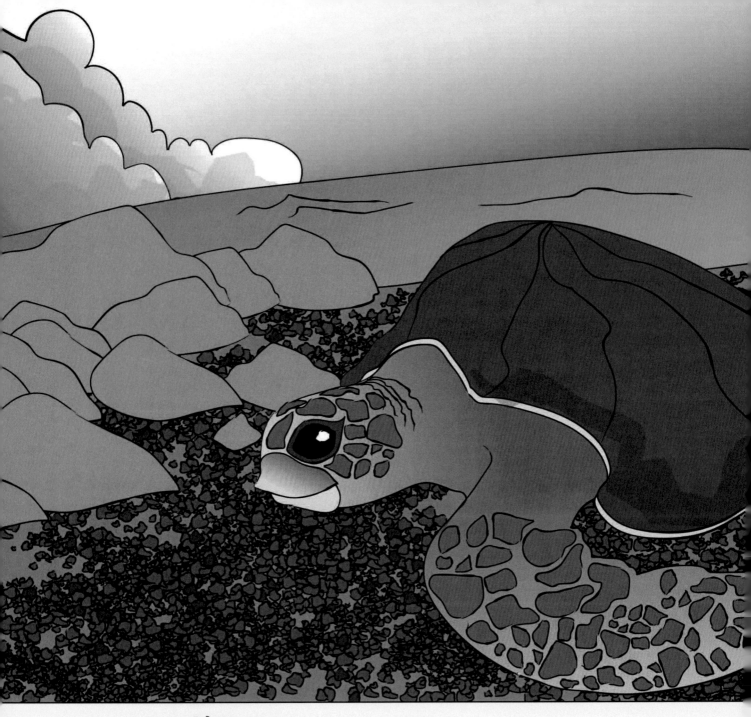

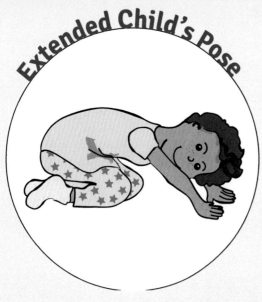

Extended Child's Pose

The **turtle** is nesting in the black sand.
Good night, turtle.

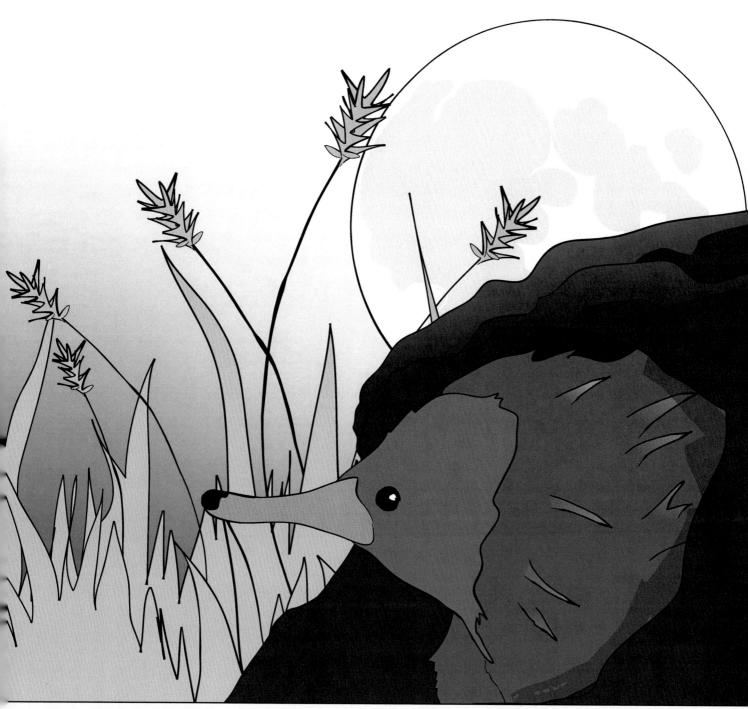

The **echidna** is burrowing in
a hollow log.
Good night, echidna.

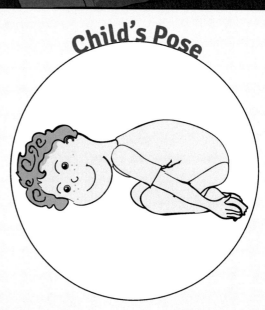

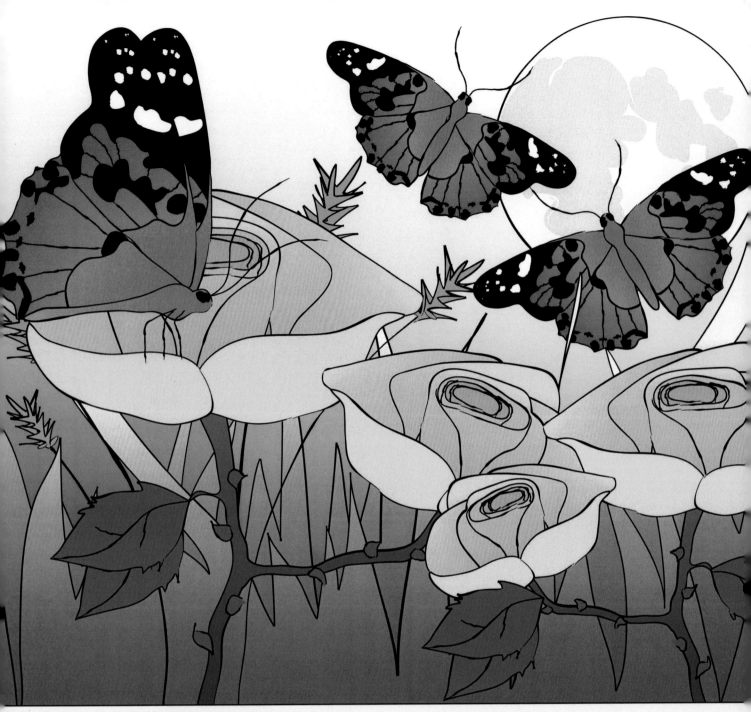

Cobbler's Pose

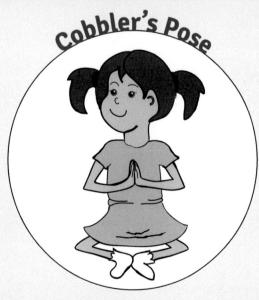

The **butterfly** is floating around the pink roses. Good night, butterfly.

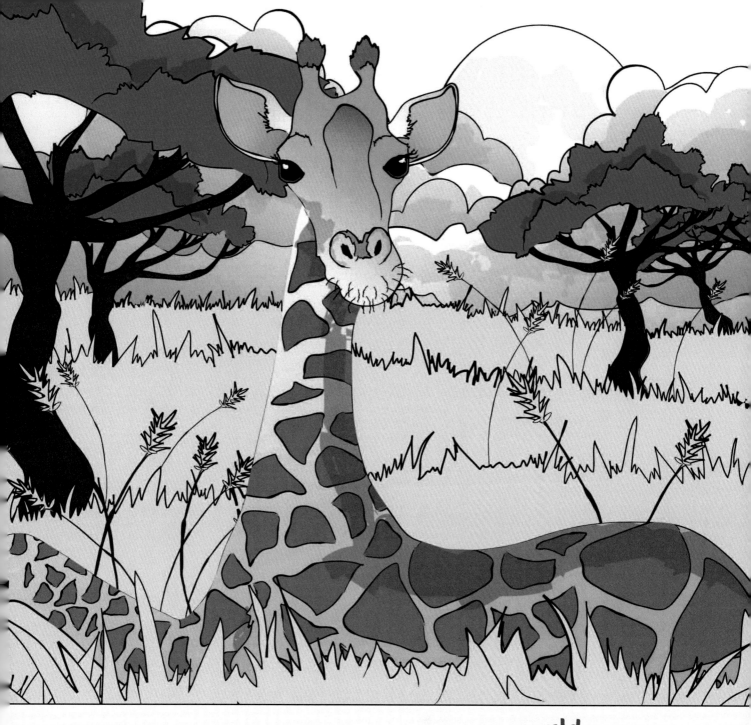

The **giraffe** is sitting down for a nap in the tall grass. Good night, giraffe.

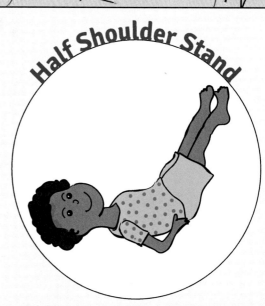

Half Shoulder Stand

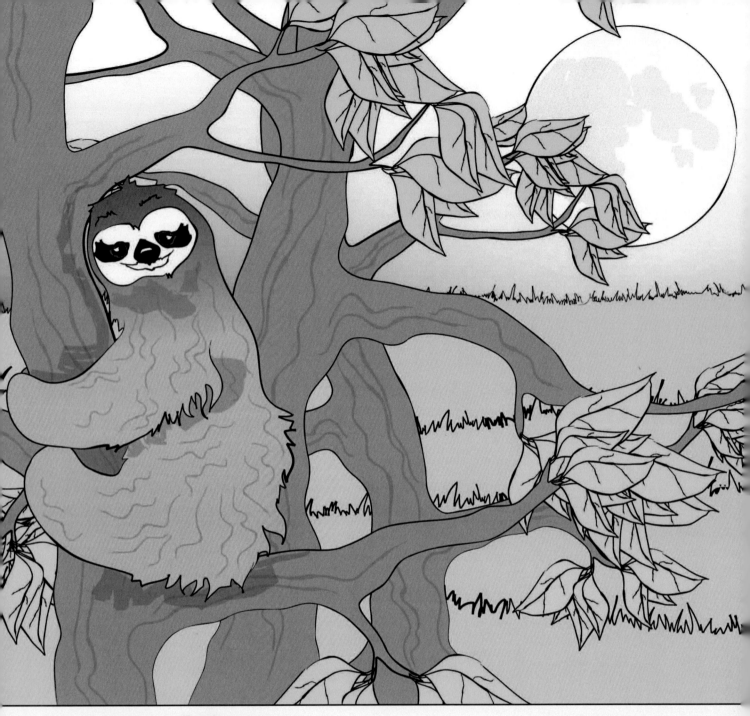

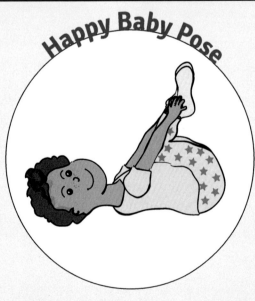

Happy Baby Pose

The **sloth** is wrapping itself around a leafy branch. Good night, sloth.

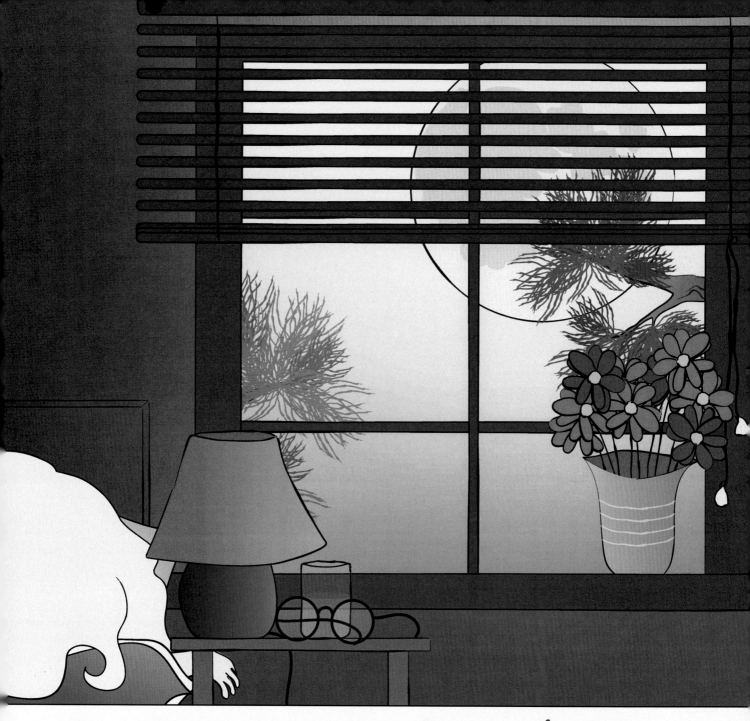

Good night, **animals**
around the world.
Good night. Sleep tight.

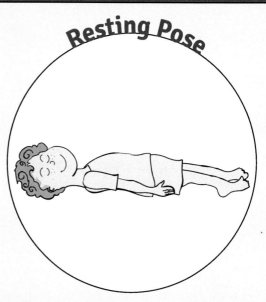

Resting Pose

The Animals Around The World

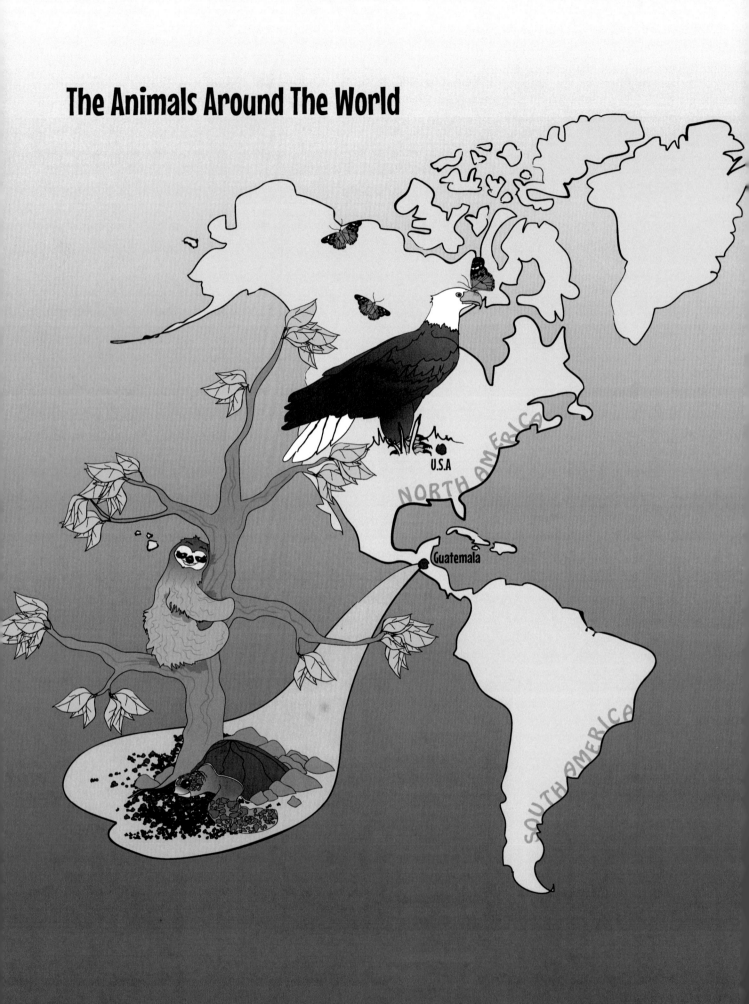

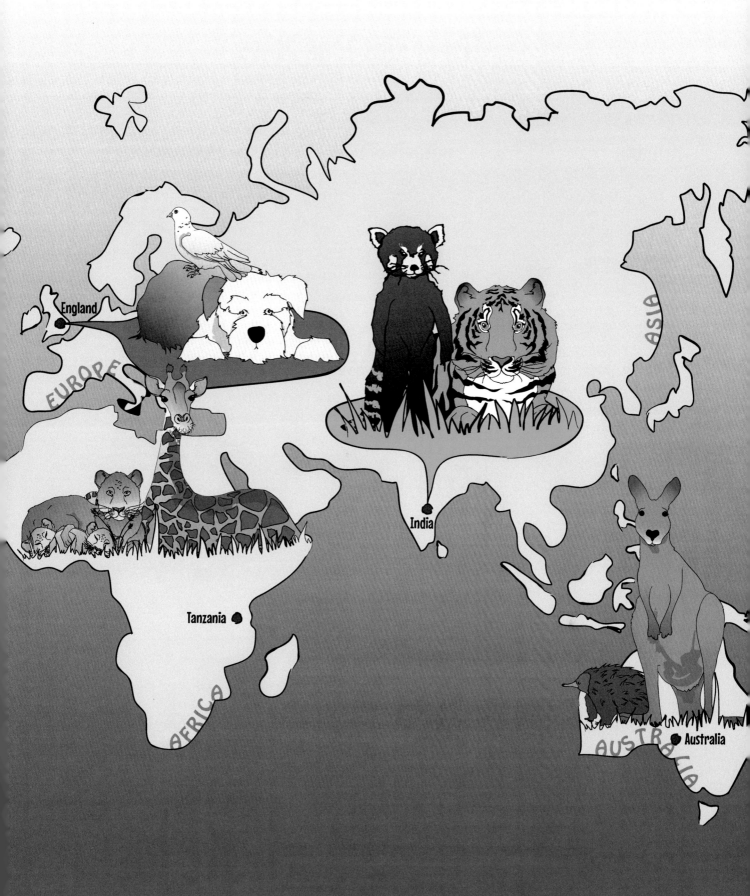

List of Kids Yoga Poses

The following list is intended as a guide only. Please encourage the children's creativity while ensuring their safety.

ANIMAL	YOGA POSE	DEMONSTRATION
1. Red Panda	Moon Salute	
2. Red Kangaroo	Kangaroo Pose	
3. Bald Eagle	Eagle Pose	
4. Bengal Tiger	Squat Pose	
5. Sheepdog	Downward-Facing Dog Pose	
6. Turtle Dove	Pigeon Pose	

ANIMAL	YOGA POSE	DEMONSTRATION
7. African Lion	Cat Pose with Lion's Breath	
8. Sea Turtle	Extended Child's Pose	
9. Short-beaked Echidna	Child's Pose	
10. Monarch Butterfly	Cobbler's Pose	
11. Masai Giraffe	Half Shoulder Stand	
12. Brown-throated Sloth	Happy Baby Pose	
13. All Animals	Resting Pose	

Kids Yoga Stories Guide

Please seek professional guidance from your pediatrician about any specific sleep questions or issues that your child experiences. Referring to recent sleep research or speaking to a sleep expert is also highly recommended.

These practical tips are based on my experience as a mom:

Use this book as a guide. The list of poses is intended as a guide only. Please encourage the children's creativity while ensuring their safety.

Put safety first. Ensure that the space is clear and clean. Spend some time clearing any dangerous objects or unnecessary items. A suitable space could be your child's bedroom or your living room. Wear comfortable clothing, and practice barefoot.

Props are welcome. Lay out a yoga mat for your child. Blankets or towels could be used in place of a yoga mat, if you are practicing on a non-slip surface. Bolsters or blocks could be used, as well. Props often help to signal yoga time, and children will associate these items with their yoga experience.

Create calming environment. Play soothing music, dim the lights, speak in a calming voice, and clean up the space to help create a peaceful atmosphere. This helps children relax their mind and bodies.

Practice a calming sequence. The kids yoga poses in this bedtime book were specifically chosen for their calming effects. The poses are also laid out in a specific sequence to invite a flow from one pose to the next. Feel free to add other animals to your family yoga experience, but try to avoid stimulating poses. Calming poses are forward bends, restorative poses, gentle twists, and some inversions.

Create a consistent ritual. Choose a regular bedtime ritual that works for your family. You might follow the Four B's each night—brush, bath, book, and bed. A massage after bath time is another great way to invite calm and connection. A consistent routine fosters trust and safety, so anyone who follows the routine—a family member or sitter—can put the child to bed with ease.

Start early. It's never too early to start a bedtime ritual. In fact, the earlier the better. The whole family benefits from healthy sleep habits. Use the same ritual, such as reading a book, before each daytime nap and nighttime sleep with children as young as newborns. Books read together in the bedroom signal sleep time.

Involve your child. Talk to your child about the bedtime ritual. Explain what you are doing and what comes next. Give them time indicators by saying things such as, "Five minutes until we brush our teeth." Then announce, "It's bath time." Be consistent and clear in your communication.

Go slow. Take your time to work through the poses in the book. Its purpose is to guide your child through unwinding from her busy day. Take your time, and help her to slow down.

Cater to your child's age. Use this Kids Yoga Stories bedtime book as a guide, but make adaptations according to the age of your child. Feel free to lengthen or shorten your bedtime journey to ensure that your children are fully engaged throughout your time together. Our recommendation is to read with children ages two to five (toddlers to early primary). Break the journey down into a couple of poses for each session if you are working with ages two to four. Add more poses or extend the ideas if you're working with children over four years old. They might make up their own stories about the animals, invent their own poses, read books about the animals, take pictures of themselves in the poses, or paint pictures of the poses and animals. Extension activities could be done during the day and not necessarily right before bedtime, depending on the energy level required for the activity.

Relax. Allow your children time to end their session in Resting Pose for five to ten minutes. Massage their feet during or after their relaxation period. Relaxation techniques give children a way to deal with stress. Reinforce the benefits and importance of quiet time for their minds and bodies. Introduce meditation (as simple as sitting quietly for a couple of minutes) as a way to bring stillness to their highly stimulated lives.

Talk together. Engage your child in the book's topic. Talk about the animals or traveling to different places so they can form meaningful connections. Also, talk about what they did that day and their plans for the next day. This helps build memory skills and makes them feel safe.

Use repetition. Feel free to repeat the bedtime sequence as many times as your child is engaged. Ask your child to say or predict the next pose in their around-the-world animal journey.

Learn through movement. Brain research shows that we learn best through physical activity. Our bodies are designed to be active. Encouraging your children to act out the animals not only allows them to have fun, but also helps them to learn about different animals and techniques for active relaxation.

Develop breath awareness. Throughout the practice, feel free to bring attention to the action of inhaling and exhaling in a light-hearted way. For example, encourage the children to take long audible exhales to imitate the sounds of the lion and tiger. Take deep breaths when you are resting in the turtle and echidna poses.

Lighten up and enjoy yourselves. A children's yoga experience is not as formal as an adult class. Encourage the children to use their creativity, and provide them time to explore the postures. Avoid teaching perfectly aligned poses. The journey is intended to be joyful and fun.

Be uplifting. Create a positive bedtime ritual that your child looks forward to each night. Talk about what your family is grateful for each day. Establish an environment where happiness is seen as something we can cultivate inside and out. Happiness then becomes a daily habit.

Connect with each other. Read and act out the book together. Whether it is two siblings or cousins, a grandparent and grandchild, or a parent and child, that connection is important. Bond with the little people in your life. Cherish the moment. Live in the present.

Be flexible. Be willing to change the bedtime ritual, depending on the needs of your child. Notice if they are particularly tired and should shorten or skip one of the bedtime routines. Or read more bedtime books if they are engaged and the books are helping to bring calm. Encourage them to select which books they would like to read before bedtime. Honor their preferences.

Be engaging. Your child will feed off your enthusiasm for the book. They will be more likely to engage in the poses if you practice them together. Enjoy yourselves. Take the opportunity to calm your own "monkey mind," as well.

Build good sleep habits for life. Your child's sleep habits will potentially affect his or her health, academic performance, and emotional well-being. Treasure these magical moments and know that you are giving your child the gift of healthy sleep habits for life.

About Kids Yoga Stories

We hope that you enjoyed your **Kids Yoga Stories** experience.

Visit our website, www.kidsyogastories.com, to:

Receive updates. For updates, contest giveaways, articles, and activity ideas, sign up for our **Kids Yoga Stories Newsletter.**

Connect with us. Please share with us about your yoga journey. Send us pictures of yourself practicing the poses or reading the story. Describe your journey on our social media pages (Facebook, Pinterest or Twitter).

Check out free stuff. Read our articles on books, yoga, parenting, and travel. Download one of our kids yoga lesson plans or coloring pages.

Read or write a review. Read what others have to say about our books or post your own review on Amazon or on our website. We'd love to hear how you enjoyed **Good Night, Animal World**.

Thank you for your support in spreading our message of integrating learning, movement and fun.

Giselle
Kids Yoga Stories

www.kidsyogastories.com
info@kidsyogastories.com
www.facebook.com/kidsyogastories
www.pinterest.com/kidsyogastories
www.twitter.com/kidsyogastories
www.amazon.com/author/giselleshardlow

About the Author

Giselle Shardlow draws from her experiences as a teacher, traveler, mother, and yogi to write her yoga-inspired children's books. This story was inspired by her passion for integrating yoga and healthy bedtime habits. She lives in Boston with her husband and daughter.

About the Illustrator

Emily Gedzyk is a world traveler, animal lover, who draws her artistic inspiration from the places she's visited and the people in her life. She hopes to continue her journeys to new, exciting places and to teach everyone she meets that it's never too early or too late to go out into the world on their own adventures, and to be kind to all creatures, big and small.

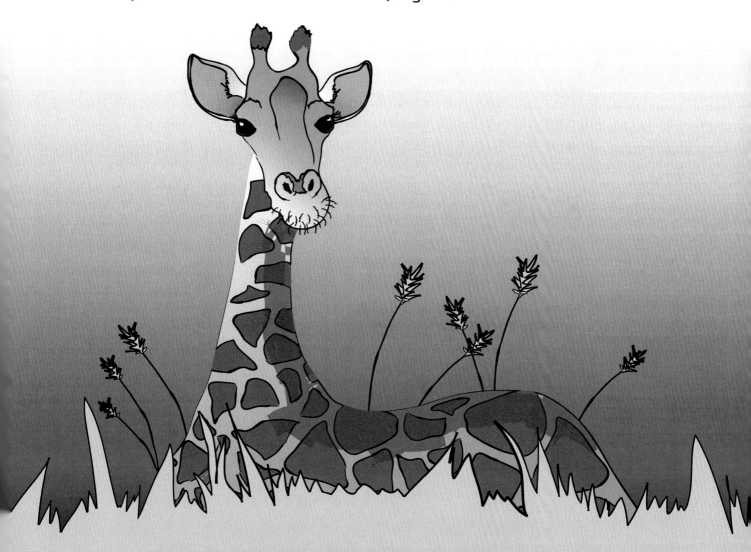

Other Yoga-inspired Books by Giselle Shardlow

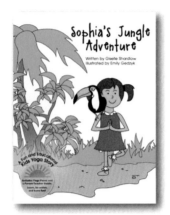

Sophia's Jungle
Adventure

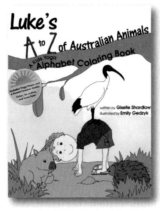

Luke's A to Z of
Australian Animals:
A Kids Yoga Alphabet
Coloring Book

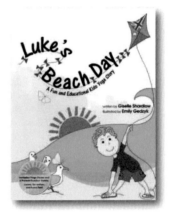

Luke's Beach Day

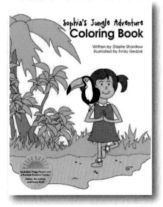

Sophia's Jungle
Adventure
Coloring Book

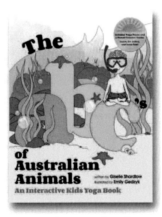

The ABC's of
Australian Animals

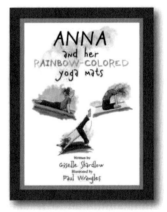

Anna and her
Rainbow-Colored
Yoga Mats

Many of the books above are available in
Spanish and eBook format.

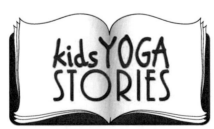

www.kidsyogastories.com

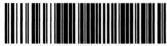
Made in the USA
San Bernardino, CA
06 September 2016